**W9-CFS-371**

# Being Vegetarian

Written for
The American Dietetic Association
by Suzanne Havala, MS, RD, FADA

## JOHN WILEY & SONS, INC.

New York • Chichester • Weinheim • Brisbane • Singapore • Toronto

This book is printed on acid-free paper. ∞

Copyright © 1996 by the American Dietetic Association.
All rights reserved
Published by John Wiley & Sons, Inc.
Published simultaneously in Canada
Previously published by Chronimed Publishing

The information contained in this book is not intended to serve as a
replacement for professional medical advice. Any use of the information
in this book is at the reader's discretion. The author and the publisher
specifically disclaim any and all liability arising directly or indirectly
from the use or application of any information contained in this book.
A health care professional should be consulted regarding your specific
situation.

Library of Congress Cataloging-in-Publication Data:

ISBN: 0-471-34661-6

Printed in the United States of America

10 9 8 7 6 5 4 3

# Being Vegetarian

**Written for The American Dietetic Association by**
Suzanne Havala, MS, RD, FADA
Suzanne Havala Nutrition Consultants, Inc.,
Chapel Hill, North Carolina

**The American Dietetic Association Reviewers:**
Ruth Carey, RD
Portland, Oregon

Winston J. Craig, PhD, RD
Andrews University
Barren Springs, Michigan

Eleese Cunningham, RD
National Center for Nutrition and Dietetics
Chicago, Illinois

**Technical Editor:**
Betsy Hornick, MS, RD
The American Dietetic Association
Chicago, Illinois

THE AMERICAN DIETETIC ASSOCIATION is the largest group of food and health professionals in the world. As the advocate of the profession, the ADA serves the public by promoting optimal nutrition, health, and well-being.

For expert answers to your nutrition questions, call the ADA/National Center for Nutrition and Dietetics Hot Line at (900) 225-5267. To listen to recorded messages or obtain a referral to a registered dietitian (RD) in your area, call (800) 366-1655. Visit the ADA's Website at www.eatright.org.

# Contents

*Part One*
# Laying the Groundwork

# Introduction

"IF YOU DON'T EAT MEAT, what do you eat?" Most vegetarians have heard that question more than once.

It's not surprising. Even though more than 12 million U.S. adults consider themselves vegetarians, a diet that takes meat off the center stage and puts it on the side (or off the plate entirely) is still sometimes misunderstood.

To a large extent, our culture determines which foods we eat and which we do not. Most Americans were raised in a meat-and-potatoes tradition, so the idea of avoiding meat—and possibly even eggs and dairy products—sparks many questions. For starters: Is a vegetarian diet healthy? Is it for everyone? Can you get all the nutrients you need? Do you have to swear off meat entirely?

The answers to these and other questions abound as we discover more and more about what constitutes a "balanced meal."

Eating well today means centering meals around foods that come from the soil—fresh vegetables, whole grains, and legumes—the backbones of a healthy diet. Meals built from these foods are a feast of colors, textures, flavors, and aromas.

Anyone can eat vegetarian—part-time or all of the time. It's just a matter of knowing how.

## What Do Vegetarians Eat?

Vegetarian diets are usually described in terms of the foods they don't include. Some vegetarians don't eat red meat, for instance, and some avoid eggs. In the truest sense, though, a vegetarian is a person who never eats meat, fish (or seafood), and poultry. Instead, vegetarians eat a wide range of foods that come from the soil, including fruits, vegetables, grains and grain products, nuts, seeds and legumes, and dried beans and peas. Some vegetarians include eggs and/or dairy products, while others avoid all foods of animal origin.

## What's in a Name?

The term "vegetarian" means different things to different people. Since vegetarian styles can vary in the extent to which they exclude animal products, most people speak of various types of vegetarian diets.

Vegetarians and their eating styles are often classified into three major types. They are:

**Lacto-ovo vegetarian.** A lacto-ovo vegetarian avoids meat, fish, and poultry but may eat eggs and dairy products, such as milk, cheese, and yogurt. Most vegetarians in the United States and Canada are lacto-ovo vegetarians.

**Lacto-vegetarian.** Like the lacto-ovo vegetarian, a lacto-vegetarian avoids meat, fish, and poultry but may eat dairy products, such as milk, cheese, and yogurt. However, unlike the lacto-ovo vegetarian, a lacto-vegetarian also avoids eggs and any foods that contain eggs or derivatives of eggs such as egg albumin or egg whites.

**Vegan.** Vegans (pronounced *vee gun*) are strict vegetarians who avoid all animal products. A vegan never eats meat, fish, poultry, eggs, and dairy products. Vegans avoid foods that contain any derivatives of these ingredients, too, such as whey, casein, and other hidden animal product ingredients. Many vegans also avoid honey, since they consider the use of honey to be exploitive of bees.

## The Vegetarian "Continuum"

Even within types, or categories, vegetarian eating patterns can differ from one another, depending upon the extent to which a person excludes animal products. For example, one lacto-ovo vegetarian may eat cheese, milk, and eggs on a daily basis, while another may eat them only occasionally—maybe a few times per month. Both people are described as lacto-ovo vegetarians, but the nutritional composition of their diets may be quite different. Some people avoid red meat but eat fish and poultry. They are sometimes referred to as semi-vegetarians or meat-restrictors. Others avoid red meat and poultry but do eat fish. At what point is someone a vegetarian, or at what point are they a nonvegetarian?

In reality, there are many variations in eating patterns—even among types of vegetarians. In this way, vegetarianism can be thought of as a continuum, ranging from an eating pattern that includes limited amounts of meat to a strict vegetarian or vegan diet and all points in between.

## The Vegetarian Continuum

| | | | | |
|---|---|---|---|---|
| Traditional American Diet | Meat Restrictor | Lacto-ovo Vegetarian | Lacto-Vegetarian | Strict Vegetarian or Vegan Diet |

Considering how widely vegetarian eating patterns can differ from one another, it may make sense to describe them by what they have in common, rather than by what sets one apart from another.

Vegetarian eating styles are planned around plant-based foods. They have as their foundation foods that come from the soil—fruits, vegetables, grains, nuts, seeds, and legumes. Foods of animal origin, if included at all, are a minor part of the diet. They are a condiment, side dish, or an ingredient in a dish, rather than the focal point of the plate.

## Vegetarian Foods Are Universal

Needless to say, vegetarian foods have been around a long time. Historically, most of the people of the world have eaten a largely vegetarian diet. Only in affluent societies such as Europe and North America, where meat and animal products have been affordable to the masses, has a diet centered around meats become traditional. In other areas of the world, people have traditions of meals that are plant-based.

## Vegetarian Traditions Around the World

Your favorite ethnic cuisine probably includes many vegetarian dishes that are native to other countries. Do you enjoy Mexican foods, such as beans and rice, bean burritos, or cheese enchiladas? What about Greek spanakopita, or spinach pie? Italian foods, such as eggplant parmigiana, spaghetti with marinara sauce, or cheese-stuffed manicotti and canneloni? How about Thai vegetable curries, Oriental vegetable stir-fries, or Indian dal? The list goes on and on.

## The Health Connection

According to survey reports, most people adopting a vegetarian-style diet today do so primarily for health reasons. They consider vegetarian eating to be part of a healthy lifestyle.

In fact, vegetarian lifestyles are associated with a decreased incidence of many chronic, degenerative diseases and conditions, such as heart disease, many types of cancer, diabetes, high blood pressure, obesity, and others. There is also decreased incidence of kidney stones, gallstones, and diverticular disease in vegetarians.

In general, people who eat vegetarian are also likely to avoid alcohol, caffeine, and tobacco, and they are more likely to exercise regularly. Good health habits such as these undoubtably contribute in great part to the good health records of vegetarians. However, the vegetarian diet itself is likely a major contributor to the health status of vegetarians.

Foods of plant origin contain many substances that help protect against disease and promote good health. Examples of these components include fiber and antioxidant nutrients such as beta-carotene, vitamins C and E, and other vitamins and minerals. Research is showing that phytochemicals in foods also play a role in disease prevention. For instance, a substance called genistein, found in soy beans, has been shown to be associated with lower rates of colon, prostate, and breast cancers. Soy foods have also been shown to lower blood cholesterol levels. Well-planned vegetarian diets are also notable for what they don't contain. Plant-based eating patterns are typically lower in total fat, saturated fat, and cholesterol.

## Concern for the Environment

Many people choose to become vegetarian as a way of contributing to the preservation of our natural resources and minimizing damage to the environment. Some are concerned that cattle grazing can cause the erosion of topsoil, and that the farms on which most food animals are raised make intensive use of our increasingly precious water supplies. Others cite problems with pollution caused by animal agricultural practices. In contrast, some feel that the cultivation of plants for direct human consumption uses much less land, water, energy, and other resources.

## An Ethical Choice

For many vegetarians, the choice to not eat animals centers on ethical beliefs. Their choice is an expression of their compassion for animals or ideas about nonviolence. Vegans take their beliefs one step further than their diet and extend their avoidance of animal products to their choices in clothing, cosmetics, and other items. As much as possible, they avoid products that have animal ingredients or that have been tested on animals.

## And the List Goes On...

Ask ten vegetarians for their reasons for being vegetarian, and you are likely to get ten different answers.

Oftentimes, there is more than one reason that a person chooses a vegetarian diet. Some religions, such as Hinduism or the Seventh Day Adventist Church, among others, advocate vegetarian eating styles. Some people simply avoid animal-based foods for aesthetic reasons—they don't like the way the foods look or taste, or they don't like the idea that meat, poultry, and fish are animal flesh. Others see their choice of being vegetarian as a way to help alleviate world hunger or make a political statement concerning the balance of power within developing nations. For still others, the choice centers on spiritual reasons.

*Chapter One*
# Nutrition Talk

MOST OF US learned about nutrition using the Basic Four Food Groups. The "Basic" Four consisted of 1) fruits and vegetables, 2) grains, 3) dairy products, and 4) meats.

The old Basic Four Food Groups model for meal planning has been retired and replaced with a more relevant tool, the Food Guide Pyramid. In contrast to the Basic Four, the Food Guide Pyramid (see page 16) demonstrates visually that grains, fruits, and vegetables are the foundation foods of a healthful diet, whether you are a vegetarian or not.

Nevertheless, generations of us have the old message permanently etched in our minds: dairy products and meats are cornerstones of a balanced eating pattern. For instance, name a good source of calcium. Most people would say milk or cheese. Which foods are high in protein? Cheese, eggs, and meat. And iron? Red meat. It can be challenging to reprogram the way we think about meals and eating.

In reality, a vegetarian eating style can provide all of the nutrients you need. No animal products are necessary. However, raised on a meat-and-potatoes dietary tradition, most of us are conditioned to think of animal products when asked to name good sources of vitamins, minerals, and other nutrients.

You may wonder where these nutrients will come from in a plant-based eating style. Let's look at some of the key nutrients.

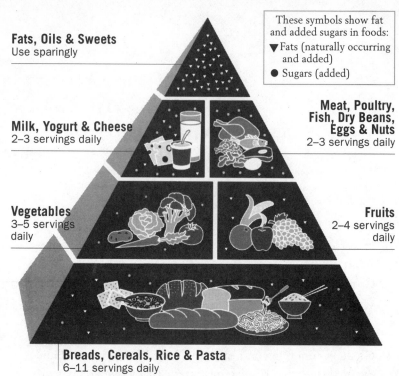

U.S. Department of Agriculture/U.S. Department of Health and Human Services, 1992.

**Fats, Oils & Sweets**
Use sparingly

These symbols show fat and added sugars in foods:
▼ Fats (naturally occurring and added)
● Sugars (added)

**Milk, Yogurt & Cheese**
2–3 servings daily

**Meat, Poultry, Fish, Dry Beans, Eggs & Nuts**
2–3 servings daily

**Vegetables**
3–5 servings daily

**Fruits**
2–4 servings daily

**Breads, Cereals, Rice & Pasta**
6–11 servings daily

## Which Foods Provide Protein?

Most of us can name animal products that are high in protein. Meat, fish, poultry, eggs, cheese, milk, yogurt, and other dairy products are rich in protein. But what about other foods? Which plant foods are high in protein?

Protein is abundant in grains and grain products, legumes, seeds and nuts, and many vegetables. These foods can provide you with all of the protein that you need. Legumes, or dried peas and beans, are especially rich in protein. Examples include pinto beans, kidney beans, lentils, garbanzo beans, split peas, black beans, and navy beans. Seeds, nuts, and nut butters are also concentrated in protein (but note that they're quite high in fat, too). If you eat a reasonable variety of plant foods each day and get enough calories to meet your energy needs, it is almost impossible for you not to get enough protein.

## Protein Powerhouses

| | |
|---|---|
| Four bean salad | Hummus |
| Vegetarian chili | Bean burrito |
| Bagel with peanut butter | Eggplant parmesan |
| Bowl of oatmeal | Navy bean soup |
| Lentil soup | Vegetarian burger |
| Vegetable stew | Bean taco |
| Vegetarian chili | Pasta with vegetables |
| Split pea soup | Vegetable paella |
| Falafel | Spanakopita |

Twenty or thirty years ago, a theory was popularized that said that in order for vegetarians to get enough protein, they had to carefully combine certain foods. The "complementary protein theory" maintained that protein from plant foods was inferior to protein that came from animal products. The idea grew from the fact that most plant foods are limited in one or more of the essential amino acids—the building blocks of protein. Therefore, the conclusion made was that plant foods had to be eaten in combinations, at the same meal, to complement their amino acid profiles and match one food that was lacking in a particular amino acid with another food that had an abundant supply of that amino acid.

The complementary protein theory was widely accepted at one time and gave many people the impression that it was risky, complicated, or tricky at best to get enough protein in a vegetarian diet. Vegetarians carefully combined beans with rice, peanut butter with bread, or added cheese or eggs to dishes in order to ensure that they met their protein needs.

Although the concerns regarding the quality of plant proteins were correct, emphasis placed on the need for conscious combining of foods was not. Combining specific plant foods at meals is not necessary. In reality, as long as you are eating enough wholesome foods to meet your calorie needs and are getting a reasonable mix of vegetables, grains, and legumes over the course of the day, you should not have any problems getting enough protein or the appropriate mix of amino acids.

At the same time, you will probably avoid the excessive amounts of protein that can be typical of the traditional

Western-style diet. A more moderate protein intake has important advantages, as you will see in the next section.

## What About Calcium?

As you know, milk is a rich source of calcium. So are cheese and yogurt. Vegetarians that include dairy foods can get plenty of calcium by eating these foods. But what if you don't eat dairy products? Which other foods contain calcium?

Vegetarians who do not eat dairy products can get plenty of calcium from plant foods. Calcium is widely distributed among a broad range of vegetables, grains, legumes, and some fruits. Some examples of foods that are good sources of calcium are green leafy vegetables such as kale, collards, mustard and turnip greens, broccoli, bok choy, dried beans, tofu that has been prepared with calcium, sesame seeds, orange juice fortified with calcium, and many others.

Calcium intakes in vegetarians that are below levels recommended in the United States do not appear to result in health problems. For instance, osteoporosis is not more common in vegetarians than it is in nonvegetarians. This may be due to better absorption and retention of dietary calcium from vegetarian diets, relating in part, to a more moderate protein content. People who consume large amounts of protein, as is typical of a traditional Western eating style, can lose more calcium through their urine.

In fact, recommendations for calcium intake in the United States are established to compensate for calcium losses due to high protein intakes. Since vegetarians have lower protein intakes, they may have lower calcium needs, as well. In countries where the diet is more plant-based, recommendations for calcium are about one-half of the amount recommended in the United States

Nevertheless, it is still important for vegetarians to eat plenty of good plant sources of calcium. Children, teens, and young women should be especially careful to include daily servings of calcium-rich foods in their diets, since their calcium needs are relatively high compared to other people. (See Chapter 7)

Also note that too much salt (or sodium), caffeine, or phosphorus can reduce the amount of calcium your body absorbs. Go easy on foods that are high in sodium such as table salt, salty snacks, processed foods, and caffeinated beverages such as tea, coffee, and soft drinks.

### Good Vegetarian Sources of Calcium

| | |
|---|---|
| Collard, turnip, and mustard greens | Blackstrap molasses |
| Broccoli | Kale |
| Bok choy | Calcium-fortified soy milk |
| Tahini | Calcium-fortified orange juice |
| Almonds | Sunflower seeds |
| Tofu processed with calcium | Dried figs |
| | Kidney beans, navy beans, and garbanzo beans |

## What About Iron?

Red meat is high in iron, right? But if you don't eat red meat, which foods provide iron?

Just like calcium, iron, too, is widely distributed in plant foods. In fact, some of the same foods that are good sources of calcium are also good sources of iron. Examples of iron-rich plant foods include dark green leafy vegetables such as spinach, kale, and collard greens, dried beans, watermelon, dried fruits, prune juice, blackstrap molasses, pumpkin seeds, sesame seeds, and many others. Vegetarians can get enough iron by eating a variety of these foods.

However, just as important as getting enough iron from foods is ensuring that the body can absorb it. Certain substances in foods can inhibit or enhance your body's ability to absorb the iron in your diet.

Vitamin C helps the body absorb iron. When you eat a food that is rich in vitamin C at a meal, it helps your body absorb any iron that is present at that same meal. Good sources of vitamin C include citrus fruits and juices, tomatoes, cabbage, strawberries, green peppers, and broccoli, to name just a few.

You probably eat vitamin C-rich foods with many of your meals and don't even realize it. Do you eat tomato sauce over spaghetti, or drink a glass of orange juice with your breakfast cereal? Do you add green peppers to a salad or have a slice of watermelon for dessert?

Just as vitamin C helps you absorb iron from foods, certain components of other foods can inhibit iron absorption. For example, tannins in coffee and tea can reduce iron absorption from a meal in half. It's a good idea to limit coffee and tea with meals.

Phytates, found in whole grains, can bind with iron and prevent its absorption as well. In some poor countries, for instance, the diet is based on low-iron grain staples that are high in phytates, with few fruits or vegetables that provide vitamin C to enhance iron absorption. This contributes to problems with iron deficiency. Other factors, such as parasites, low protein intakes (with resulting low blood hemoglobin levels), and a high consumption of unleavened flat breads (leavening decreases phytate levels) are also contributors to iron deficiency in poor countries.

Malabsorption of iron is more likely to be a problem in cultures where poverty prevents people from obtaining a variety of foods. When food choices are varied, however, inhibitors and enhancers of iron absorption generally offset each other—in other words— they balance each other out. In Western countries, vegetarians are not more prone to iron deficiency than are nonvegetarians. Nevertheless, it's still important that you eat a variety of iron-containing foods.

## Iron-Rich Vegetarian Foods

| | |
|---|---|
| Soy nuts | Swiss chard |
| Spinach | Watermelon |
| Lentils | Sesame seeds |
| Kale | Pinto beans |
| Raisins | Iron-fortified cereals |
| Broccoli | Prune juice |
| Blackstrap molasses | Bean burritos |
| Bok choy | Figs |
| Garbanzo beans | Bean chili |

## And Zinc?

Studies show that vegetarians usually consume enough zinc, although meeting recommended dietary intakes of zinc can be a challenge for vegetarians as well as nonvegetarians. Generally, legumes, nuts, seeds, and whole grains are good plant sources of zinc. Wheat germ is particularly rich in zinc. Adding a sprinkle of wheat germ to a bowl of oatmeal, over steamed vegetables, or on top of a casserole, can help to boost the zinc content of the meal.

### Vegetarian Zinc Boosters

| | |
|---|---|
| Tofu | Wheat germ |
| Pumpkin seeds | Cashews |
| Peanut butter | Pecans |
| Baked beans | Millet |
| Tahini | Black beans |
| Tempeh | Split peas |
| Miso | Lima beans |
| Hummus | Pinto beans |
| Sunflower seeds | Fortified breakfast cereals |
| Lentils | |

## Where Do You Find Vitamin D?

Vitamin D is the sunshine vitamin. Why? Because your body manufactures its own vitamin D when your skin is exposed to sunlight. You can actually get all of the vitamin D you need this way.

Few foods are naturally good sources of vitamin D. Liver happens to be rich in vitamin D, since the liver is a storage site in the body for vitamin D, but vegetarians don't eat liver. In the United States, milk and milk products have been fortified with vitamin D for many years. In a sense, if you drink milk, then you get a supplement of vitamin D. This safeguard was put into place when it was recognized that some people were not receiving adequate exposure to sunlight and were suffering from vitamin D deficiencies. One consequence of vitamin D deficiency is rickets, a childhood disease in which the bones are soft and deformed.

Vegetarians who drink milk and eat other dairy products

generally do not have to worry about getting enough vitamin D. But what about vegans and other vegetarians who consume no dairy products? Should they be concerned about vitamin D?

If you avoid dairy products and you are not regularly exposed to direct sunlight, then the best advice is to check with your physician or a registered dietitian to determine whether or not you need a vitamin D supplement. Those who are most likely to have problems with inadequate exposure to sunlight are people who are housebound, or those who are dark-skinned, or live in very northern latitudes or in smog-filled cities (also see Chapter 7).

Fortunately, the body can store vitamin D that is produced in the summer months for use during the winter months when sun exposure may be lessened. For adequate vitamin D production, you need about 20 to 30 minutes of summer sun on hands and face two to three times per week. If a vitamin D supplement is indicated, however, then care should be taken not to exceed 100 percent of the Recommended Dietary Allowance, since excessive amounts can be toxic. If you're taking a calcium supplement for bone health, you may be getting vitamin D as well since it is added to many calcium supplements.

## Which Foods Contain Vitamin B12?

Vitamin B12 is needed in very small amounts in the diet—less than 3 micrograms per day. It wouldn't seem hard to get such a small amount of a vitamin, and it isn't—for most people. Vitamin B12 deficiency takes a long time to develop, but once it does, it can cause irreversible nerve damage. In everyone, vegetarian or not, vitamin B12 deficiency is more likely to be caused by a lack of intrinsic factor, a substance that must be present in the stomach in order for vitamin B12 to be absorbed, than from a dietary deficiency.

Vitamin B12 is produced by microorganisms in the intestines, or guts, of animals as well as humans. In humans, however, it is thought to be produced beyond the site of absorption in the intestines. Therefore, we can't rely on being able to utilize the vitamin B12 that is produced in our bodies.

All animal products contain vitamin B12 so a vegetarian who

eats eggs, milk, cheese, or other dairy products can get all of the vitamin they need from these foods. Your need for vitamin $B_{12}$ is so small, that even the occasional consumption of animal products is likely to provide you with the vitamin $B_{12}$ you need.

In some parts of the world, where sanitary practices are not as well-developed as in Western cultures, vitamin $B_{12}$ can be obtained from non-animal sources. Microorganisms that produce vitamin $B_{12}$ are present in the soil. Foods grown in soil, if not washed thoroughly, may contain vitamin $B_{12}$ in the soil still clinging to them. A sip of water taken from a mountain stream may contain vitamin $B_{12}$-producing microorganisms as well.

However, not many Westerners grow their own food or drink from mountain streams, and health practitioners would not recommend that anyone get their vitamin $B_{12}$ through these routes. In our modern, sanitary world, our produce is washed clean at the supermarket, and our water is chlorinated.

Therefore, vegans—those vegetarians who never eat foods of animal origin—need to ensure that they have a reliable source of vitamin $B_{12}$ in their diets. It isn't difficult to do, but it is important. What are some reliable sources of vitamin $B_{12}$ for vegans? A supplement is one option. Look for the word "cyanocobalamin." This is the form of vitamin $B_{12}$ that is physiologically active for humans. In other words, it is the form that we most readily utilize.

Other options include foods that have been fortified with cyanocobalamin. Some commercial breakfast cereals are fortified with vitamin $B_{12}$. Read package labels to check. Also note that manufacturers sometimes change the ingredients in their products from time to time. So if you find a product that contains vitamin $B_{12}$, check the label again from time to time to be sure that it has not been removed.

Commercial soy milks are also increasingly being fortified with vitamin $B_{12}$. So are vegetarian burger patties and other vegetarian specialty foods available in supermarkets and natural foods stores. One brand of nutritional yeast, Red Star T6635, is another good source and can be found in natural foods stores.

What about spirulina, miso, nutritional yeast (other than Red Star T6635), tempeh, and sea vegetables? These are foods often available in natural foods stores that are thought by some to be good sources of vitamin $B_{12}$. They may even list "vitamin $B_{12}$" on their nutrition labels. In fact, they are not reliable sources. Some of these foods list vitamin $B_{12}$ on their labels but, in reality, they contain a mix of cyanocobalamin and other forms, or analogs, of the vitamin. The laboratory process used to measure these foods' vitamin $B_{12}$ contents does not differentiate between cyanocobalamin and other forms of the vitamin. Nutrition scientists caution that the majority of the vitamin $B_{12}$ present in these foods may be analogs and, therefore, not utilized by humans. The analogs may actually compete for absorption with the cyanocobalamin that we need.

The bottom line: look for the word "cyanocobalamin" on food labels or ingredient lists to be sure that the food product you are buying is a reliable source of vitamin $B_{12}$. The other option: take a cyanocobalamin supplement. About two and a half micrograms per day is enough to meet recommended needs for most teens and adults.

### Good Vegetarian Sources of Vitamin $B_{12}$

Red Star Nutritional Yeast T6635

Vitamin $B_{12}$-fortified soy milk

Vitamin $B_{12}$-fortified breakfast cereals

Vitamin $B_{12}$-fortified vegetarian burger patties

Other vegetarian specialty foods fortified with vitamin $B_{12}$

## Should I Take Vitamin and Mineral Supplements?

Most healthy vegetarians don't need to take vitamin or mineral supplements, although there may be exceptions. For instance, as noted earlier, vegans need to be sure to have a reliable source of vitamin $B_{12}$ in their diets. If they don't, then they should take a vitamin $B_{12}$ (cyanocobalamin) supplement. And people who don't drink milk or eat other dairy products might need a vitamin D supplement if they also have inadequate exposure to sunlight.

If you have doubts about the adequacy of your food choices, consult a registered dietitian or your health care provider for his or her opinion. Even when a supplement is needed, care may need to be taken not to exceed recommended amounts, since some vitamins and minerals can be toxic at high levels.

Also, nutrients interact with each other, and imbalances can be created when too much of a single vitamin or mineral is taken. For instance, zinc and iron interact with each other. If you receive too much zinc from a supplement, you may deplete your iron stores. It's always best to check with your health care provider before taking a supplement of any single nutrient. Generally, multivitamin and mineral supplements are recommended, as opposed to single-nutrient preparations.

Keep in mind that supplements cannot make up for a poor diet. In fact, it's best to depend on getting the nutrition that you need from whole foods, rather than from supplements. There may be essential substances in whole foods that have not yet been identified and are not present in vitamin and mineral supplements. By taking care to eat a nutritious, varied diet instead, you help to ensure that you'll get what you need.

*Part Two*
# Making the Switch to the Vegetarian Way

*Chapter Two*
# Making the Switch

SOME PEOPLE MAKE THE SWITCH to a vegetarian eating style overnight. Others prefer to take a more gradual approach. There is no best way to make such a lifestyle change. Do what feels comfortable for you.

If you choose to take the gradual approach, you might begin by simply cutting down on the amount of meat you eat at meals and eating more meatless meals throughout the week. When you include meat with meals, make it a minor ingredient in a dish, rather than the focal point of the plate. Some other tips for getting started are:

**Make a list of all of the meatless dishes you already enjoy.** Make a conscious effort to fix these often.

**Browse through some vegetarian cookbooks and look for recipes or meal ideas that sound appealing.** Bookstores are loaded with good vegetarian cookbooks, and your local library also stocks them.

**Take a trip to a local natural foods store and experiment with a few products.** You might find an interesting new convenience item (pinto bean flakes and quick-cooking grains are two examples). Another good place to begin is in the natural foods aisle of your neighborhood supermarket, where some of these specialty products are beginning to appear.

**Try "meat alternative" products made with soy and other vegetable and grain ingredients.** These can be good transition foods as you reduce your meat intake, since they're familiar and can be used in the same ways as their real meat counterparts. They're quick and convenient, too. Examples include vegetarian burger patties, hotdogs, breakfast meats, and similar products.

## Eating Well the Vegetarian Way

Planning a healthful vegetarian diet is easier if you keep the following points in mind:

**Think variety.** Include a range of plant foods, including fruits, vegetables, whole grain breads and cereals, and legumes, or dried beans and peas. Build your meals around these foods—the possibilities are endless. Think pasta tossed with steamed vegetables, vegetarian multi-bean chili over rice, bean burritos and tacos, vegetable stir-fries, and more.

**Get enough calories to meet your energy needs.** When you include a reasonable variety of foods and adequate calories, it's likely that you'll meet your nutritional needs as well.

If you are underweight and having trouble gaining weight, eat more frequently. Include snacks between meals. Add some higher calorie foods to your eating pattern. You may need to replace some bulky, low-calorie vegetables with starchy, more calorie-dense choices such as potatoes, squash, peas, or beans. For instance, rather than filling up on a tossed salad, choose a hearty bean and pasta soup instead.

If you are overweight and reducing your fat and calorie intake to help lose weight, be extra careful to choose nutrient-dense foods and to limit sweets and junk foods. When you restrict calories, there is less room in the diet for foods that provide little nutrition in exchange for their calories.

**Limit your intake of sweets and fatty foods.** These foods may take the place of more nutritious food choices. While there's room in most peoples' diets for an occasional treat, too many empty-calorie foods will make it difficult to meet your nutritional needs. Soft drinks and french fries are vegetarian foods, but an eating pattern built around foods such as these does little to promote good health.

**If you are vegan, remember to include a reliable source of vitamin B12 in your diet.** See page 24 for examples.

*Chapter Three*
# Setting Up Shop
*The Vegetarian Kitchen*

REMEMBER WHEN you could only find rice cakes and tofu at your local health food store? Times have changed.

Today, it's likely that your neighborhood supermarket has everything you need to stock a vegetarian kitchen. In fact, the bulk of most vegetarians' food needs can be found in any neighborhood supermarket—fruits and vegetables (fresh, frozen, and canned), breads, cereals, pasta, rice and other grains, beans and peas (dried or canned), lentils, and so on. And brands that used to be found only in natural foods stores are increasingly finding space on supermarket shelves, so you can pick up your soy milk and vegetarian chili mix at the same time that you buy your orange juice and canned beans.

If you can't find what you want in your supermarket, however, try your local natural foods store. Many communities now have natural foods stores that handle large volumes of food and can offer competitive prices on specialty items. Some of the larger stores offer products such as soy milk, vegetarian soups, chili, packaged foods, and so on at prices that are significantly lower than what mainstream supermarkets can offer. It pays to comparison shop.

On the other hand, you should also know that you don't have to eat specialty products—which can be relatively expensive—in order to be a vegetarian. It's a matter of personal preference.

Some people find that as they grow more comfortable and familiar with vegetarian meals, they begin to experiment with more ethnic dishes that make use of exotic or unfamiliar ingredients. Since these foods may not be commonplace in our culture, they are more likely to be found in natural foods or specialty stores than in your neighborhood supermarket. Examples of such foods are Asian sea vegetables, tamari, tempeh, Indian frozen entrées such as mutter paneer or curried vegetables, Middle Eastern tahini, and exotic grains such as quinoa, spelt, and amaranth.

## Stocking Your Cupboards, Fridge, and Freezer

If you are new to a vegetarian lifestyle, you may find that a little extra structure in the beginning—writing weekly menus and keeping a shopping list—is helpful.

The shopping lists* that follow can be adapted to suit your own food preferences or buying habits. (Vegans will want to avoid any egg or dairy products listed; lacto-vegetarians will avoid egg products listed.) Take them with you when you shop, or just use them to peruse for ideas. There are separate lists for foods that are likely to be purchased weekly, monthly, or less often.

## Weekly Shopping List

Buy these items weekly, since they are perishable:

### Fresh Fruit (especially locally-grown fruits in season)

| | |
|---|---|
| apples | mangoes |
| apricots | nectarines |
| bananas | oranges |
| blueberries | papayas |
| cantaloupe | peaches |
| cranberries | pears |
| grapefruit | pineapples |
| grapes | plums |
| honeydew | strawberries |
| kiwi | watermelon |
| lemons | others |
| limes | |

---

*Shopping lists are adapted from *Simple, Lowfat & Vegetarian* by Suzanne Havala (Vegetarian Resource Group, 1994) with permission from the publisher.

## Prepared Fresh Fruits

fresh juices: orange, grapefruit, tangerine, apple cider, and others

packaged, cut fruits
chilled, bottled tropical fruit salad, mango or papaya slices, or pineapple chunks

## Fresh Vegetables
### (especially locally-grown in season)

asparagus
bean sprouts
beets
bell peppers
bok choy
broccoli
brussels sprouts
cabbage
carrots
cauliflower
celery
collard greens
corn

cucumbers
kale
kohlrabi
leeks
mustard greens
onions
potatoes
salad greens (leaf lettuce, romaine, etc.)
sweet potatoes
tomatoes
zucchini
others

## Prepared Fresh Vegetables

fresh vegetable juices: carrot, carrot spinach, beet
packaged, cut vegetables

packaged, washed salad greens
fresh herbs: basil, dill, mint, rosemary, sage, thyme, and others

## Breads (especially whole grain)

English muffins
French bread
Italian bread
multigrain bread
oatmeal bread
pita pockets

pumpernickel
rye
sourdough
whole wheat
others

## Rolls (especially whole grain)

hard rolls
hoagie rolls
kaiser rolls

onion rolls
others

## Bagels (limit egg bagels)

blueberry

cinnamon raisin

mixed grain

oat bran

onion

plain

poppyseed

pumpernickel

rye

sesame seed

whole wheat

others

## Other Bread Products
### (especially whole grain)

corn tortillas (not fried)

flour tortillas

fresh pizza crusts

low-fat muffins

## Fresh Pasta (limit pasta made with egg yolks)

## Fresh Deli Items

four-bean salad

fresh fat-free salad dressings

fresh marinara sauce

fresh pizza (cheeseless or
  vegetarian)

fresh salsa

others (ask to see recipes;
  look for low-fat or nonfat
  items)

## Fat-free or 1% Milk

## Low-Fat or Nonfat Yogurt (soy or dairy)

## Low-Fat or Nonfat Cheese (soy or dairy)

## Eggs (limit yolks) or Refrigerated Egg Substitute

## Fresh Tofu (look for low-fat)

## Also need:

_____

_____

_____

_____

_____

_____

_____

## Monthly Shopping List

These items can be purchased less often, since they can keep longer in the cupboard or freezer:

## Cupboard Staples

### Canned Goods

beans (canned or dry): vegetarian baked beans (look for fat free), garbanzo, black beans, black-eyed peas, kidney, navy, split peas, lentils, and others
bean salad (in jars)
soups: lentil, vegetable, vegetarian split pea, tomato
spaghetti sauce
tomato sauce and pasta
refried beans (without lard)

applesauce (bottles and individual servings)
fruits: peaches, pears, mandarin orange sections, grapefruit sections, cranberry sauce, fruit cocktail, apricots, pineapple
vegetables: green beans, peas, carrots, asparagus, corn, tomatoes, and others
sloppy joe sauce

### Dry Items

pasta (limit pasta made with egg yolks)
dry cereals (especially whole grain): raisin bran, shredded wheat, bran flakes, and others
cooked cereals (especially whole grain): oatmeal, rye, multi-grain, and others
whole wheat flour
wheat germ

whole grain bread, pancake, and all-purpose mixes
other whole grain mixes
rice: basmati, brown, wild, and others
barley
bulgur wheat
couscous (look for whole grain)
textured vegetable protein (bulk or mixes)

### Soup Mixes

### Vegetable Oil Spray

### Snacks and Treats

rice cakes and popcorn cakes
popcorn (low-fat or fat-free)

flat breads, bread sticks, and matzo

pretzels
bean dip (fat-free)
baked tortilla chips
crackers (especially whole grain)

cookies (look for low-fat, whole grain)
canned pumpkin and fruit pie fillings

**Soy Milk (in aseptic packages or a mix; also rice milk or other nondairy)**

**Tofu (in aseptic packages)**

**Condiments**
maple syrup
jams and jellies
salsa
blackstrap molasses
nonfat or reduced-fat salad dressings

reduced-fat mayonnaise (regular or egg-free)
vinegar: red wine, rice, cider, raspberry, balsamic, etc.
mustard
ketchup
chutney

**Spices and Vegetable Bouillon**

**Mineral Water, Seltzer Water, and Club Soda**

**Bottled Fruit Juices**

**Bottled Vegetable Juices**

**Herbal Teas**

**Vegetable Oils (use sparingly; buy small bottles)**

**Dried Fruits**
apples
apricots
dates
figs

mixed fruits
prunes
raisins

**Nuts and Seeds (use sparingly)**
peanut butter and almond butter
almonds: slivered, whole, sliced

sunflower seeds
tahini
walnuts

**Also need:**

_____

_____

_____

_____

_____

_____

_____

_____

_____

## Freezer Staples

### Frozen Bagels (limit egg bagels)

### Frozen, Plain Vegetables
| | |
|---|---|
| broccoli | peas |
| spinach | soup mix |
| corn | mixed vegetables |
| green beans | stir-fry mix |

### Frozen Fruit
| | |
|---|---|
| blueberries | raspberries |
| strawberries | mixed berries |

### Frozen Fruit Bars

### Sorbet

### Juice Concentrates
| | |
|---|---|
| blends (pineapple-orange, orange-peach, etc.) | orange juice |
| | grapefruit juice |
| lemonade | |

### Frozen Waffles (whole grain, low-fat)

### Frozen Muffins (whole grain, low-fat)

### Frozen Egg Substitute

## Specialty Foods (choose low-fat)

| | |
|---|---|
| tempeh | vegetarian hot dogs |
| vegetarian burger patties | frozen entrées |

**Also need:**

_____

_____

_____

_____

_____

_____

_____

_____

_____

_____

## Tips for Savvy Shoppers

**It pays to shop with a list in hand.** Keep a running tally of what you need. Post it on your refrigerator or nearby so that when you see you are running low on an item, you can add it to your list. Then be sure to take the list with you when you shop. Keeping a list will save you the time and frustration of going back for something you forgot. More importantly, shopping from a list can help you save money and avoid impulsive purchases—often sweets and fatty junk foods.

**Avoid shopping when you are hungry** and are more likely to make impulsive purchases. If those impulsive purchases were bananas and black beans, there might not be a problem. Most people, however, find that cookies, chips, and ice cream end up in their baskets. Have a piece of fruit or a few crackers if you need to before you leave home.

**Get into the habit of reading food labels.** Check the fat and fiber content of foods. Look at the list of ingredients. Compare similar products to see which is the best nutritional value.

## The Weekend Cook

Now that you have the staples in your kitchen, take a little time—20 minutes to an hour—to fix a few foods that you can eat over the next several days. This might become a weekend tradition—taking time out when your schedule is less harried to prepare some items that you may not have time to fix later in the week.

Here are some ideas to get you started. Add some of your own to the list.

**Fruit salads:** use seasonal fruits for interesting combinations such as cantaloupe balls with blueberries, strawberries, and bananas, or peaches and blueberries. Toss with lemon, orange, or lime juice to prevent browning.

**Mixed green salads:** spinach and strawberries are a delicious combination

**Coleslaw:** try it with a low-fat vinaigrette dressing

**Vegetable salads:** such as four bean, carrot raisin, or marinated fresh vegetables

**Soups:** bean, lentil, split pea, gazpacho, potato leek

**Chili:** use several types of beans; add corn for color

**Whole-grain pancake and waffle batter:** keeps for a day or two in the refrigerator, but store in freezer for longer periods

**Hummus (chick-pea spread):** add some chopped vegetables such as red bell peppers, scallions, or grated carrots

**Pasta dishes:** Tofu-stuffed shells or manicotti, or vegetable lasagna

**Cooked rice:** a big batch; it reheats quickly and can be eaten with leftover vegetables or chili

## Fix and Freeze Foods

Many of the foods listed above can be prepared in large batches. Set aside enough for a few days and freeze the rest. Pasta dishes, muffins, soups, and chili freeze well and can keep for several weeks. Leftover pancakes and waffles can also be frozen. Reheat frozen pancakes in the microwave oven; waffles can be popped into the toaster.

## Easy Snack Ideas

Draw from the foods you have on hand for quick and easy snacks and mini-meals on the run:

Pretzels

Fruit shakes and smoothies

Popcorn

Whole-grain crackers

Frozen juice bars with peanut butter

Dairy or soy yogurt

Bagels

Fresh vegetable sticks with salsa dip

Muffins

Fresh fruit

Hummus on pita bread

Dried fruit and fruit leather

Baked potatoes topped with lentil soup or chili

Soup

Chili

Vegetarian pizza, with or without cheese

Bean burritos

Bean tacos

Hot cereal with fruit

Dry cereal and milk (dairy or nondairy)

Dinner leftovers

*Chapter Four*
# Planning Meals the Vegetarian Way

USE THE DAILY VEGETARIAN FOOD GUIDE, adapted from USDA's Food Guide Pyramid, that follows to assist you in planning your meals if you are new to the vegetarian way. If you are a veteran vegetarian, use the guide to evaluate your current eating style and help identify areas that might need improvement.

Adults should eat at least the minimum number of servings indicated for each food group. Pregnant women, athletes, or anyone who needs more calories should choose extra servings from each of the food groups. A good rule of thumb for most healthy people is to eat according to your appetite. It also merits repeating: vegans should remember to include a reliable source of vitamin $B_{12}$ in their diets.

## Make the Most of Your Food Choices
When making choices from the food guide, pay special attention to the following points:

**Choosing Breads, Cereals, Rice, and Pasta.** The goal is to aim for a minimum of six servings a day, of which at least half are whole grains.

It's fine to enjoy refined grain foods such as English muffins, most bagels, and French bread for the sake of variety. However, whole-grain products should predominate your choices, since they are such good sources of fiber. Whole grains also have a higher vitamin and mineral content than refined grains, which lose nutrients in processing. Whole grains are a good source of zinc, for example. When you do buy refined grain products, choose those that have been enriched.

Expand your horizons. Try some foods that may be new to you. The world of grains is much bigger than whole-wheat bread and brown rice. Have you tried millet, quinoa (pronounced *keen wah*), spelt, or amaranth? You might also enjoy jasmine or basmati rice. Grains are versatile. They can form the base of a meal, such as couscous (a tiny, round, quick-cooking semolina product) with mixed vegetables, pasta with beans, or a rice casserole. They also work well as an added ingredient. Add a handful of barley or bulgur wheat (rolled, cracked wheat), for instance, to thicken soups and stews. Millet goes well with chili. Wheat germ is a good topping on casseroles and broiled tomatoes. Stuff cabbage rolls with garbanzo beans and cooked rice.

Mix several grains together when cooking. Multigrain cooked cereal is delicious, for instance. If you have a bread machine or enjoy baking bread from scratch, it can be fun to experiment with different blends of grains and develop your own "signature" recipe.

Some grains are available in "quick-cooking" form. These are fine to use and can usually be found in whole-grain form as well. These grains may have been parboiled and cut into smaller pieces to increase their surface area and decrease cooking time.

When buying pasta, look for varieties that are made without eggs. There is a wide variety available now, and they are also lower in cholesterol than pastas made with eggs.

When choosing breakfast cereals, look for those that have been fortified with vitamins and minerals. Vegans should read labels and look for cereals with vitamin $B_{12}$, cyanocobalamin.

**Choosing Vegetables.** The goal is four or more servings per day.

Fresh, frozen, and canned varieties of vegetables are all nutritious options.

It may cost more to buy peeled and cut vegetables, but for people who are short on time, the convenience of buying pre-prepared fresh vegetables such as washed, mixed salad greens or peeled baby carrots may make the difference between eating vegetables with a meal or not. For single people or small families, buying smaller quantities of prepared vegetables can actually be

# Daily Vegetarian Food Guide

| Food group | Suggested daily servings | Serving sizes |
|---|---|---|
| **Breads, cereals, rice, and pasta** | 6 or more | 1 slice whole grain or enriched bread<br>1/2 bun, bagel, or English muffin<br>1 tortilla<br>1/2 cup cooked cereal (oatmeal, rye, mixed grain)<br>1/2 cup cooked rice, millet, quinoa, bulgur, barley, and other grains<br>1/2 cup cooked pasta<br>1 oz. dry cereal |
| **Vegetables** | 4 or more | 1/2 cup cooked or chopped, raw<br>1 cup raw, leafy<br>3/4 cup vegetable juice |
| **Fruits** | 3 or more | 1 medium piece fresh fruit<br>3/4 cup fruit juice<br>1/2 cup canned or cooked fruit |
| **Legumes and other meat substitutes** | 2 to 3 | 1/2 cup cooked dry beans or peas<br>4 oz. tofu or tempeh<br>8 oz. soy milk or soy yogurt<br>1 1/2 oz. soy cheese<br>2 Tbsp. nuts or seeds<br>2 Tbsp. peanut butter<br>3 oz. vegetarian burger patty or 1 vegetarian hotdog<br>1 egg or 2 egg whites<br>1/4 cup egg substitute |
| **Dairy products (optional)** | up to 3 servings daily | 1 cup milk or yogurt<br>1 1/2 oz. natural cheese<br>2 oz. processed cheese |
| **Fats, oils, and sweets** | Go easy on these foods | Oil, margarine, mayonnaise, salad dressings<br>Candies |

cost-effective if it results in less spoilage and waste.

When buying frozen vegetables, keep in mind that added sauces can increase the fat content considerably.

Canned vegetables may be rinsed with water to reduce the salt content if desired.

Be sure to include plenty of dark green, leafy vegetables, such as kale, collard, and mustard greens; broccoli; and bok choy. They are rich in calcium, iron, vitamin A, and folic acid.

Include vitamin C-rich vegetables such as tomatoes, cabbage, green peppers, and broccoli. They also help your body absorb iron.

Make it a habit when you come home from grocery shopping to spend 20 to 30 minutes washing, peeling, and chopping fresh vegetables. Store them in plastic bags or containers in the refrigerator until you need them. They will be ready to steam, sauté, or add to salads or stir-fries. You'll save precious time later when you prepare meals and may not be in the mood for extensive meal preparation.

When you pass through the produce section at the supermarket, take a few extra minutes to check out some of the vegetables that may be unfamiliar to you. Take a chance and try something new. You may even find some new favorites.

Enjoy seasonal vegetables. Stop at roadside stands and farmers' markets during the growing season to find fresh, locally-grown vegetables.

**Choosing Fruits.** The goal is to aim for a minimum of three servings per day.

Fruit juice is fine, but don't let it replace fresh fruit. Fresh fruit can be a good source of fiber, where fruit juice is not.

Enjoy a wide variety of fruits. Keep several kinds of fruit in your home at all times. Include those that are rich in vitamin C, such as grapefruit, oranges, watermelon, strawberries, and kiwi. When you buy fruit juices, choose those with vitamin C added, unless they are already high in vitamin C, such as orange and grapefruit juices.

When you are in the produce section of your supermarket, take some extra time to shop for fresh fruit. Experiment with something you have never tasted—perhaps an exotic fruit such as mango or papaya. You may find some new favorites.

If fresh fruit seems to be sitting too long in your refrigerator or fruit bowl, cut it up and make a fruit salad. Try different combinations of fruits, such as melon cubes with berries or peaches with blueberries. Add some chopped figs to a winter salad of apples, pears, and oranges or to a bowl of hot cereal.

Wash and cut fresh fruit into pieces and store it in an airtight container on the top shelf of the refrigerator, where it will be easily spotted the next time you are looking for a quick and easy snack. Toss the fruit with a little lemon juice to prevent browning. Eat a few pieces with breakfast, or add some to your lunch or dinner plate as a garnish.

Buy seasonal fresh fruits. Make it a habit to stop at roadside stands or farmers' markets for fresh, locally-grown fruits. Picking fruits in season can be a fun family activity that can result in everyone eating more of them.

Vegans or anyone looking for an easy source of calcium should remember that calcium-fortified orange juice is available.

**Choosing Legumes and Other Meat Substitutes.** The goal is to aim for two to three servings per day.

Beans are fiber superstars. One cup of cooked beans such as pintos or black beans contains about 16 grams of fiber! In addition to being high in fiber, vitamins, and minerals, legumes are versatile and delicious. Use dried beans (and peas) in soups, vegetable stews and vegetarian chili. Cooked, mashed beans make a good sandwich filling. Mashed pinto beans or black beans work well in bean burritos, tacos, and nachos, and they make a good dip for fresh vegetable sticks, too.

Dried beans and peas can be prepared from their dried form by soaking overnight before cooking. However, if this process is inconvenient for you, it's fine to use canned beans. If you wish to reduce the salt that is added to most canned beans, simply rinse the beans with water before using them.

Visit local ethnic food marts to see a range of choices that you may not find in your neighborhood supermarket. Indian grocery stores, for example, usually stock an amazing array of lentils in colors you may not have known existed.

Tofu is now available in reduced-fat varieties. The regular

variety is moderately high in fat. Tofu is actually quite versatile. Did you know that tofu can be used to make puddings, sauces, dips, quiche, and pie fillings? See Chapter 6 for more information.

Soy milk, like tofu, is available in reduced-fat varieties. It can also be found fortified with vitamins and minerals, including vitamin $B_{12}$ and calcium. Soy milks vary in flavor; most have a slightly "beany" aftertaste which many people find quite pleasant. You may want to experiment with several brands to find your favorite.

Soy milk is also versatile and can be used measure for measure in place of cows milk in recipes. It's delicious on breakfast cereals or by the glass. Try using soy milk with fresh fruit to make nutritious "smoothies."

Nuts and seeds are high in fat, so you may want to use them sparingly. This includes nut and seed butters, such as almond butter and tahini.

Vegetarian burger patties and other meat alternative products can be convenient and nutritious alternatives to their meat counterparts. Many of the products available now are fat free or very low in fat, and some provide several grams of fiber in a serving. Read nutrition labels on packages and comparison shop. Also note the sodium content and choose products that are lower in sodium if you're watching your sodium intake.

Soy yogurt and soy cheese are available in natural foods stores. They tend to be high in fat, although manufacturers are creating more low-fat products all the time. Check food labels; choose low-fat products if they're available. If you are using full-fat varieties, use them in small quantities or only occasionally to help keep your total fat intake low.

**Dairy Products.** Milk, cheese, yogurt, and other dairy products are optional in a vegetarian eating pattern since other foods can supply the nutrients found in dairy products.

For those who choose to eat dairy products, up to two to three servings per day are suggested (or up to four for teens and pregnant women).

While dairy products are a good source of calcium, they are low in iron and devoid of fiber. Too much dairy in a vegetarian diet can displace other foods that provide needed fiber and other nutrients.

Choose low-fat and nonfat dairy products to help keep your total fat and saturated fat intakes low.

**Eggs.** Eggs are optional for vegetarians. If you choose to eat them, limit yolks to four per week to help control your dietary cholesterol intake.

**Fats, Oils, and Sweets.** Limit fats such as margarine, oils of all types, mayonnaise, salad dressing, butter, cream cheese, and other fatty spreads. Your overall eating pattern should be low in total fat, even if fats come from plant sources.

Limit sweets and other "empty-calorie" foods that return few nutrients for the calories they provide. These foods may take the place of more nutritious foods. Many sweets are also high in fat, such as cake, pie, and ice cream.

**Alcohol.** For vegetarians and nonvegetarians alike, alcoholic beverages such as beer, wine, and distilled spirits should be limited to two drinks per day for men and one drink per day for women. One drink equates to a 12-ounce beer, a 5-ounce glass of wine, or 1.5 ounces of 80-proof distilled spirits. Alcohol is a concentrated source of calories and, like many sweets, is devoid of nutrients.

*Chapter Five*
# Menu Plans
*Simple and Delicious*

VEGETARIAN MEALS CAN BE EASY to plan and prepare. Old pros may draw from supplies they have on hand and plan meals as they go, day to day. Other people like to plan ahead, sketch out a menu a week at a time, and buy groceries accordingly. Do what works best for you.

The sample menus that follow can be used to get you started if you are new to a vegetarian way of eating, or you might just refer to them to get new ideas for meals. They are only suggestions; your own food choices may reflect different food preferences or meal schedules.

The menus are planned according to the Daily Vegetarian Food Guide described in Chapter 4. They are designed for adults and average about 1,800 calories per day; some individuals may need more or fewer calories and will need to make adjustments accordingly.

The actual nutritional content of the menus will vary, depending upon your specific food choices and whether or not fortified foods are used. Aim for variety and quality in your food choices so that over time, your needs for all nutrients will be met. For instance, a low calcium intake on one day might be balanced out by a high calcium intake on another day.

The menus that follow are also planned without animal products, to make them versatile enough for any vegetarian to use. You may choose to add or substitute animal products, depending upon the type of vegetarian eating style you choose. If you are a vegan, remember to include a reliable source of vitamin B$_{12}$.

## Sample Seven Day Menu

### Day 1

### Breakfast
1 cup oatmeal with cinnamon, 2 tablespoons raisins, and
    2 tablespoons wheat germ
1 cup soy milk
2 slices whole wheat toast with jelly
3/4 cup orange juice

### Lunch
1 cup lentil soup
Mixed green salad with tomatoes and reduced-fat
    dressing
Carrot and green pepper sticks with salsa
1 whole grain muffin
Water with fresh lemon

### Dinner
1/2 cup marinated bean salad (kidney, garbanzo, and
    green beans)
1 cup pasta tossed with 1 teaspoon olive oil, garlic, and
    basil with a sprinkling of nutritional yeast
1/2 cup stewed tomatoes and okra
1/2 cup steamed broccoli with lemon juice
1 slice Italian bread
1/2 cup fresh fruit salad
Flavored seltzer water

### Snack
Bagel with jam

# Day 2

## Breakfast

2 raisin bran muffins
1/2 cup flavored soy yogurt
1/2 grapefruit
3/4 cup cranberry-orange juice

## Lunch

1 cup vegetable soup
Eggless egg salad (tofu salad) sandwich on rye bread
1/2 cup vinaigrette cole slaw
1 tangerine
Water with lemon

## Dinner

Vegetarian black bean burger on whole-grain bun with
   lettuce, tomato, pickles, ketchup, and mustard
Baked potato wedges
1/2 cup orange-glazed cooked carrots
Baked apple with maple syrup and cinnamon
Hot herbal tea

## Snack

3 cups popcorn
Flavored seltzer water

# Day 3

## Breakfast
2 slices eggless French toast with maple syrup
Sliced banana
3/4 cup orange juice

## Lunch
1 cup vegetarian many-bean chili over 1 cup steamed rice
1/2 cup cooked kale with sesame seeds
1/2 cup steamed corn
2 peach halves
Water with lemon

## Dinner
2 tofu-stuffed manicotti
1/2 cup steamed green beans
1/2 cup parsleyed potatoes
Chunk of Italian bread
1/2 cup nondairy ice cream
Water with lemon

## Snack
1 cinnamon raisin bagel
1/2 cup apple juice

# Day 4

## Breakfast

3/4 cup scrambled tofu
2 slices whole wheat toast with jelly
1/2 cup hash brown potatoes
1/2 cup orange juice

## Lunch

1 cup split pea soup
Sandwich with chick-pea spread and shredded carrots on
    multigrain roll
Tomato slices
1 slice banana bread
Water with lemon

## Dinner

Mixed baby greens salad with mushrooms, red onions, and
    balsamic vinaigrette dressing
1 cup ratatouille over 1 large slice corn bread
1/2 cup steamed cauliflower
1/2 cup orange and grapefruit sections
Water with lemon

## Snack

Sliced pear

# Day 5

## Breakfast
1 ounce bran flakes with 1 cup soy milk
1/2 cup sliced strawberries
1 English muffin with jelly
1/2 cup orange-pineapple juice

## Lunch
Spinach salad with 2 teaspoons vinaigrette dressing
Small cheeseless pizza with vegetable toppings
1 large apple
Water with lemon

## Dinner
1 cup black bean soup with chopped onions
1 1/2 cups vegetable paella
Cucumber and tomato salad
Whole-grain roll
Slice of watermelon
Water with lemon

## Snack
2 oatmeal cookies
1 cup soy milk

# Day 6

## Breakfast

1 cup seven-grain hot cereal with 2 teaspoons brown
sugar and 1/4 cup chopped dried fruit
1 cup soy milk
Fresh orange wedges

## Lunch

1 bean burrito with salsa
1 bean soft taco
Carrot and green pepper sticks
Slice of cantaloupe
Flavored mineral water

## Dinner

1 cup lentil rice pilaf
1 baked sweet potato with brown sugar and fresh lime
juice
3/4 cup cooked collard greens
2 whole-grain bread sticks
Baked pear
Water with lemon

## Snack

1 cup flavored soy yogurt

# Day 7

## Breakfast
2 whole-grain waffles with maple syrup
1/2 cup fruit salad
3/4 cup orange juice

## Lunch
1 cup potato leek soup
Baked bean sandwich on whole wheat toast
1/2 cup steamed broccoli
1/2 cup soy rice pudding
Water with lemon

## Dinner
Chick-pea-stuffed cabbage rolls
1/2 cup stewed tomatoes
1/2 cup boiled potatoes
Whole-grain roll
12 grapes
1 cup orange juice

## Snack
1/2 cup cinnamon applesauce
2 graham crackers

*Chapter Six*
# Working with Recipes

ARE YOU LOOKING FOR RECIPES that don't use eggs or milk? Having trouble finding an acceptable alternative to a favorite meat-containing recipe?

There are many good vegetarian cookbooks at bookstores and libraries, and you can find other recipes in vegetarian magazines. However, don't overlook your nonvegetarian cookbooks and favorite family recipes. You might be surprised to learn how easily many nonvegetarian recipes can be adapted to exclude such common ingredients as cheese, milk, eggs, and meat.

Some of the substitutions that follow work better in some recipes than in others. You'll need to experiment to find those that work best.

In some cases, you won't notice any difference at all between the traditional recipe and one in which a substitution has been made. Other times, the quality of the finished food product— the flavor or texture, for instance—may be slightly different. This isn't necessarily undesirable. The food may still look and taste good. Sometimes, however, it may be necessary to adjust your expectations about how a particular food will look, feel, or taste. A muffin made with banana or applesauce instead of egg may be chewier, for instance.

## Egg Replacers
Have you ever noticed how every recipe for muffins, cookies, or quick breads in traditional American cookbooks calls for eggs

(and usually milk and butter)? You would think that without eggs, we couldn't make some of these favorite recipes. Not true.

To replace one egg in recipes, you can use one of the following suggestions:

> ➤ Half of a small, ripe, mashed banana. This works best in muffin, pancake, or bread recipes, especially those in which you would not mind a banana flavor.
> ➤ 1/4 cup of tofu blended with the liquid ingredients in the recipe
> ➤ 1/4 cup applesauce or other puréed fruits such as apricots and prunes, or canned pumpkin
> ➤ 2 tablespoons of cornstarch or arrowroot
> ➤ Commercial egg replacer (sold in most natural foods stores). It's a mixture of potato starch, flour, and leavening and can be used in almost any recipe calling for eggs or egg whites, including meringue.
> ➤ About 1/4 cup of mashed potatoes or cooked oatmeal. This works well in vegetarian burger or loaf recipes in which egg would ordinarily function as a binder.
> ➤ Mashed or finely chopped firm tofu can be used in place of egg to make mock egg salad for sandwiches or a filling for stuffed tomatoes. Mashed tofu can also be combined with seasonings and scrambled as a replacement for scrambled eggs.

## Meat Replacers

Textured vegetable protein (TVP) can be used in place of ground meats in such recipes as chili, tacos, sloppy Joes, casseroles, or spaghetti sauce. Made of soy protein, TVP granules absorb the fluid in recipes and acquire the chewy consistency of meat. It's available in bulk or in boxed mixes in most natural foods stores.

Tofu or tempeh can be used in place of meat in many recipes. Either can be crumbled, cubed, grilled, stir-fried, or baked. Firm tofu holds its shape better than soft tofu.

Seitan, a wheat gluten product, can also be used in place of meat in many recipes. Seitan mixes can be purchased at natural foods stores or it can be found ready-made in the refrigerator section of the store.

Vegetarian burger patties can be used as they are or crumbled and used in place of ground meat in recipes.

Meat stuffing in such recipes as cabbage rolls or stuffed peppers can be made using combinations of foods such as beans, rice, nuts, raisins, or chopped vegetables. The meat can be left out of traditional recipes for chili and some soups, and extra beans can be used in its place. Try making vegetarian chili with a combination of beans, such as garbanzo, kidney, pinto, and black beans for an appetizing and tasty effect.

## Gelatin Replacer
Gelatin is made from animal byproducts such as bones and hooves. Instead of regular gelatin, you can use kosher gelatin, which is made from a sea vegetable. Look for it at natural foods or kosher stores.

## Dairy Product Replacers
Vegans can use soy margarine in place of regular vegetable oil margarines, which contain dairy product derivatives such as whey, skim milk solids, or casein.

Vegans can use soy cheese and soy yogurt in place of those products made from milk.

Soy milk can be used measure-for-measure in place of cows milk in most any recipe.

Nondairy frozen desserts can be used in place of ice cream and sherbet. Many nondairy frozen dessert products are made from rice milk, soy milk, or fruit juices.

Soft tofu can be blended with other ingredients to make shakes or smoothies, dips, and sauces and can replace the dairy products ordinarily used to make these foods.

*Part Three*
# Beyond the Basics

*Chapter Seven*

# Vegetarian Diets for All Ages

## Vegetarian Diets for New Moms (and Moms-to-Be)

Vegetarian eating styles can be safe and healthful if you are pregnant or breast-feeding. However, for all women—vegetarian or not—this is also a time when nutritional needs are especially high. Nutritional needs are increased to meet the needs of a growing baby and to accommodate the changes taking place in your body. Therefore, it makes sense to make this a time when greater attention and care is paid to eating well.

Women need about 300 calories per day more during pregnancy as compared to nonpregnant women. When you are breast-feeding, you need about 500 calories per day more than before you became pregnant. In light of how much higher needs are for vitamins, minerals, and other nutrients during this time, the increase in energy needs is actually relatively small. That makes it even more important to plan carefully for a nutritious diet.

Keep the following advice in mind:

**Take note of your weight gain during pregnancy.** The pattern of weight gain is different for different women, but some general observations apply to all.

Most women can expect to gain about two to four pounds during the first trimester. Weight gain begins to increase after that—typically a pound a week in the second and third trimesters. The ideal weight gain for a full-term pregnancy is 25 to 35 pounds. However, a woman who begins her pregnancy underweight should gain as much as 28 to 40 pounds, and a woman who begins her pregnancy overweight should only gain 15 to 25 pounds.

Most women can let their appetites be their guides to how much and how often they need to eat. But if you are having trouble gaining weight, look at the types of foods that you are eating and the frequency of your meals and snacks. It may be necessary to plan more meals throughout the day, or you may need to include more high-fat foods during these months.

**Getting enough protein is usually not a concern for vegetarians during pregnancy.** If you're getting enough calories to support a reasonable weight gain, and eating a variety of foods, you should get all of the protein you need. Soy products, dried beans and peas, and grains are all good sources of protein and should be part of your varied eating pattern.

**Calcium is needed for your baby's bone and tooth development.** Your body becomes more efficient at absorbing calcium from your food when you are pregnant, so if your calcium intake is somewhat low, your body will compensate by absorbing more. Nevertheless, the childbearing years are also the years in which women are accumulating bone mass themselves, so it's wise to make sure that you have plenty of calcium in your diet.

Aim for four or more servings of calcium-rich foods per day when you are pregnant. Refer back to page 19 for a list of good sources. If you think you aren't getting enough calcium from your foods, check with your health care provider about taking a calcium supplement.

**Vitamin D is needed to help the body absorb calcium.** Since dairy products are fortified with vitamin D, vegetarians who drink milk or eat cheese have a food source of the vitamin. However, since vitamin D is not usually found in foods eaten by vegans, pregnant vegans should be aware that they may need a supplement if they do not have adequate exposure to sunlight. (See page 21, Where Do You Find Vitamin D?)

**The need for iron increases during pregnancy** to accommodate the increased maternal blood volume and for the baby's blood supply. If a woman's iron status is low, the body compensates by absorbing dietary iron more efficiently; absorption is also dramatically increased during the third trimester of pregnancy. Nevertheless, if iron intake is low, it can cause a pregnant woman to become anemic. It's a challenge for most pregnant women—vegetarians and nonvegetarians alike—to meet their increased iron needs and may require an iron supplement. Check with your health care provider about the recommended dosage, and be careful not to exceed it. Too much iron can interfere with zinc absorption, and supplements can cause constipation.

**Vitamin B$_{12}$ needs are also higher during pregnancy,** so vegans need to be sure that they have a reliable source. It's also important if you plan to breast-feed to have enough vitamin B$_{12}$ stored so that your breast milk will supply enough of the vitamin for your baby. (See page 22, Which Foods Contain Vitamin B$_{12}$?)

**Folic acid needs are greatly increased during pregnancy.** Research shows that consuming enough folic acid before and during early pregnancy can decrease the risk of neural tube defects in the fetus. Folic acid is the "man-made" form of folate, a B-vitamin. Folic acid is found in fortified grain foods including bread, pasta, flour, cereals, and rice, and in supplements. Vegetarians tend to get more folate and folic acid from their food choices than do nonvegetarians. Good sources of folate are dark green leafy vegetables, whole grains, nuts, and legumes. Oranges are also a good source. Many health care providers recommend that pregnant women and women trying to conceive take a folic acid supplement to be sure they are getting enough.

**Pay attention to including good sources of zinc in your diet.** Recommendations for zinc during pregnancy are slightly higher than for nonpregnant women. Good sources of zinc include whole grains, nuts, seeds. and legumes. (See page 20, And Zinc?)

## Constipation and Morning Sickness

Constipation and morning sickness are common complaints for many women during pregnancy. Here are some tips that may make you more comfortable:

Although vegetarians tend to have high intakes of fiber, constipation can still be a problem due to hormonal changes taking place and increased pressure from the baby. Be sure to drink plenty of liquids—eight cups or more—and to eat fiber-rich whole grains, fruits, vegetables, and legumes.

Walking or any form of moderate exercise can also help relieve and prevent constipation.

Help relieve morning sickness by eating smaller, more frequent meals. Five or six meals or snacks per day, rather than two or three large meals, is preferable. Try not to let yourself get too hungry between meals, since that can aggravate feelings of nausea.

Keep crackers beside your bed and nibble on a couple before you get out of bed in the morning.

Sit upright after meals, rather than lying down.

Avoid greasy or fatty foods. These foods take longer to digest and can aggravate feelings of nausea.

Follow your nose and stomach in planning meals. If a food does not appeal to you or if the smell makes you queasy, just avoid the food for now. You may be able to tolerate it again in a few weeks. In the meantime, choose the most nutritious foods of those you can tolerate.

## Feeding Vegetarian Kids

The ideal first food for all children is breast milk. In cases where breast-feeding isn't possible or chosen, commercial baby formulas are an appropriate substitute. Formula-fed infants being raised on vegan diets can use commercial soy formulas designed for infants in place of milk-based varieties. Also note:

➤ Because breast milk doesn't contain much vitamin D, breast-fed infants may need a vitamin D supplement, especially if exposure to sunlight is limited and if mom's diet is lacking in vitamin D.

➤ After 4 to 6 months of age, infants' iron needs increase. Breast-fed infants (vegetarian and nonvegetarian alike) require a source of iron, either from iron-fortified cereal or from an iron supplement. Formula-fed infants should already be receiving an iron-fortified formula, but may also require additional iron from another source at this time.

➤ Regular soy milk should never be used in place of commercial soy formulas designed for infants. Soy milk does not contain the proper mix of nutrients to be used as the sole source of nourishment for a baby.

A vegan baby that discontinues breast-feeding before one year of age should be given a commercial soy formula for infants. After one year of age, fortified soy milk should be given until about the age of 6 years. Many commercial brands are fortified with vitamins and minerals and are available in supermarkets and natural foods stores. Other vegetarian infants can follow standard guidelines for introducing dairy products. Cow's milk should not be given to children younger than 12 months of age.

Vegetarian eating styles can be adequate and healthful for children of all ages. However, young children have nutritional needs that are high due to rapid growth and development. Therefore, once table foods have lessened the need for breast milk or formula, care should be taken to ensure that your children eat enough calories from a variety of foods.

Vegetarian diets—especially vegan ones—can be bulky or filling. Fruits, vegetables, grains, and legumes are high in fiber and low in fat. Meals can make a child full without providing many calories, so it's important to give children frequent opportunities to eat. Offering snacks between meals can help to boost calorie intake. Monitoring your child's growth is the best way to ensure that enough calories and nutrients are being consumed.

And while adults may want to limit their own fat intakes for health reasons, it may be appropriate to include some higher fat foods in a young child's diet as an added source of calories. Avocado, peanut butter and other nut butters, seeds and seed butters such as tahini, for example, can be added to foods to help increase calories at meals. Refer to the resource list at the end of this book for additional help with planning vegetarian meals for young children.

## Healthy Snacks for Kids

| | |
|---|---|
| Peanut butter sandwich | Dried fruit |
| Vegetarian pizza | Popcorn |
| Dairy or soy yogurt | Bagels |
| Bean soup | Fresh fruit |
| Bean tacos or burritos | Frozen juice bars |
| Pretzels | Fruit smoothies |

## Feeding Older Vegetarian Kids

Older children and teens have fewer problems with the bulkiness of vegetarian eating, but parents may still have concerns about whether their kids are eating right. Older children and teens may eat on the run. They may frequent fast food restaurants with their friends or prefer soft drinks and french fries to broccoli and whole grains. If you have a vegetarian child, keep the following tips in mind:

**Children learn by example.** By modeling good eating habits yourself, you'll help set the stage for your child's good eating habits.

**Involve your child in meal planning activities.** Children that help shop for groceries and assist with simple meal preparation tasks at home are more likely to show an interest in eating foods served at mealtime.

**Keep plenty of nutritious, quick foods on hand at home and make them visible.** Fresh vegetable sticks with a bowl of salsa for dipping and fresh fruit cut up into bite-sized pieces or made into a fruit salad are good snacks to have on hand. Keep them on the top shelf of the refrigerator. A tub of hummus also makes a good dip for pita wedges or carrot sticks. Four-bean salad and marinated vegetable salads are also favorites.

**Keep some convenience foods on hand for quick, no-fuss meals or snacks.** Low-fat, vegetarian microwave soup cups are fast and nutritious. Hot cereals "in a cup" are also available. Hummus, baked beans, and low-fat cottage cheese mixed with minced vegetables make good sandwich fillings to have on hand. Pinto bean flakes and black bean flakes are available, too. Add water and heat them in the microwave. They make great fillings for burritos and tacos or toppings for vegetarian nachos.

## Vegetarian Diets for Older Adults

Vegetarian eating patterns can be healthful for people of all ages, and there may be some added advantages for older adults. As people age, conditions such as obesity, high blood pressure and diabetes become more common. Many people complain of digestive system problems such as constipation, hemorrhoids, and diverticulosis. When vegetarian diets are well planned, they can be high in fiber and low in fat, which can help control or alleviate these disorders.

However, other factors affect the nutritional needs of older adults, as well. As we age, our ability to digest, absorb, and retain nutrients from our food may diminish. In the case of vitamin $B_{12}$, health experts recommend that older adults get most of their vitamin $B_{12}$ either from foods fortified with this vitamin, such as breakfast cereals, or from supplements. Older people tend to need fewer calories than younger people, too, due to a gradual decline in the rate of metabolism. If food intake also declines, it follows that a person's intake of vitamins, minerals, and other nutrients will also decrease. That makes it even more important for older adults to make their overall food choices nutrient-dense and to limit "empty calorie" foods such as many sweets and fatty foods. Regular exercise and plenty of fluids are also important.

## Chapter Eight
# Tips for Eating Out

BECAUSE MORE PEOPLE—vegetarian or not—want to order meatless meals when they go out to eat, restaurants are offering many more vegetarian options on their menus. When you are eating out, keep the following tips in mind:

Big cities usually have at least a couple of vegetarian restaurants. These are sure to have lots of options from which to choose, whatever your specific preferences. Vegans, especially, will typically find plenty of menu items made without eggs, dairy products, and honey. Check the local phone book for listings.

Many ethnic restaurants serve delicious, traditional vegetarian dishes. Chinese restaurants usually offer numerous options for vegans. Mexican, Italian, Spanish, Indian, Greek, Thai, Middle Eastern, and Ethiopian restaurants also serve many interesting vegetarian dishes.

If a menu item contains meat or another animal product that you prefer to avoid, the cook may be able to modify it to suit your needs. Don't hesitate to ask your waiter if an item can be altered. For instance, if the special for the day is angel hair pasta with marinara sauce and shrimp, ask if the same dish can be prepared without the shrimp, or ask if the cook can make a pasta primavera with the angel hair pasta instead.

If in doubt, before you order, ask about how the dish is prepared. Is cheese melted on top? Will sour cream be served on the side? If the dish is prepared with animal products that you would rather avoid, ask that they be left out.

Look for some of the following vegetarian dishes* when you eat out:

## Restaurant Type—Choose:

**Pizza** Vegetarian pizza—try adding pineapple; also try your pizza without cheese—it's good!

**Fast Food** Vegetarian burgers, bean burritos, bean soft tacos, or bean tostadas with or without cheese, pancakes, muffins, biscuits, baked potato with vegetable toppings, and salad bar. In restaurants without veggie burgers, just ask for a regular burger or cheeseburger minus the meat—ask for extra lettuce, tomatoes, onions, and pickles.

**Italian** Lentil soup, minestrone soup, pasta e fagioli (pasta with beans), pasta primavera, pasta with marinara sauce, vegetable lasagna, cheese manicotti, or baked ziti

**Mexican** Bean burritos, bean tacos, chalupas, gazpacho, cheese enchiladas, spinach burritos, spinach or cheese quesadillas, bean nachos, chile rellenos, vegetable fajitas

**Indian** Dal, vegetable curries, raitas, idli or dhoka (steamed bean and rice cakes), vegetable samosas, palak panir (spinach and cheese), mutter panir (garden peas with cheese), vegetable pakoras

**Chinese** Vegetable soup, hot and sour soup, vegetarian spring rolls and egg rolls, pot stickers (steamed vegetable dumplings), Chinese salads, mixed Chinese vegetables, broccoli with garlic sauce, steamed greens, vegetable lo mein, dishes made with tofu (bean curd) or seitan (wheat gluten)

**American** Cooked or dry cereals with skim milk, pancakes and waffles, fruit, vegetable plates, grilled cheese and tomato sandwiches, meatless Reuben sandwich, baked potato, vegetable soup

**Middle Eastern** Hummus, tabouli, falafel sandwiches, stuffed grape leaves, babaganoush, vegetarian stuffed cabbage leaves, spinach turnovers

---

*Note that some of these dishes can be high in fat, especially when whole milk dairy products are used or foods are fried.

# When You Travel

Whether you are traveling by land, sea, or air, vegetarian meals are usually available. Your options will vary depending upon the carrier and the specific circumstances of your trip.

## If you travel by air...

Most airlines offer vegetarian meals; many airlines even differentiate between vegan and lacto-ovo vegetarian diets. At the time you make your reservation, ask if a snack or meal will be served on your flight. If so, then request the type of vegetarian meal you prefer. Most airlines require a 24-hour notice of special meal requests.

If you happen to change your flight schedule after making the initial reservation, be sure to check to make sure that your special meal request was transferred to the new reservation. Regardless of the circumstance, it pays to confirm your special meal request the day before your flight.

Many airlines also offer a fruit plate in lieu of a regular meal, for times when you might prefer a lighter meal. Also, on overseas flights, ethnic-style vegetarian meals are often available, to accommodate the food preferences of people from other cultures. For instance, Asian-style or Hindu vegetarian meals might be available, with or without egg and dairy products. Try one of these special meals for a change of pace!

Despite the best of plans, sometimes special meals "miss their flight." If you find you are without your vegetarian meal, you may want to take a regular tray and eat what you can from it. If that is unacceptable to you, then ask your flight attendant for crackers, fruit, or other snacks that might be available.

Carrying your own snacks, when possible, is also a great option.

## If you travel by land...

Vegetarian entrées are served on most trains in the United States, Canada, and throughout Europe, but options may depend upon the length of the trip and the class of service. Also, while lacto-ovo vegetarian menu items might be available, vegan options may be more difficult to find.

In some cases, vegetarian entrées are part of the regular menu;

in other cases, you will need to place a special request. Some carriers require a 48-hour notice for special meal requests. Inquire about your options at the time you make your reservation.

If options are limited, think about whether regular menu items can be altered to make them suit your needs. For example, could a sandwich be made without the meat? Could several side dishes be put together on a plate to make a meal?

If no meal service is offered on your trip, or if options are limited, think about packing your own food to take along. A few ideas include nonperishable, portable items such as bagels, peanut butter sandwiches, small, aseptically-packaged boxes of soy milk or fruit juice, bags of dried fruit, fresh fruit, and slices of whole-grain, homemade quick bread. These foods work well when your mode of transportation is a car or bus, too.

## If you travel by sea...

Cruise ships are well-known for extravagant food service, and vegetarian choices typically abound. Some ships include vegetarian items on their regular menus, and most ships will make your food to order if you ask. If you have concerns, you can also ask the cruise line to mail you sample menus and information about meals before or at the time you make your reservation.

Since cruise ships often serve meals buffet-style, it can be easy to pick and choose from a wide array of foods and piece together a great vegetarian meal.

*Chapter Nine*
# Where to Get Additional Help

MAKING LIFESTYLE CHANGES—such as making the switch to a vegetarian eating style—takes time and energy. It's helpful to know where to go for support and resources to assist you in your efforts. Here are some tips to help you begin:

## Look Locally

Local vegetarian societies are a good place to start for support and to network with other vegetarians who live in your community. Many groups meet monthly and sponsor potluck dinners where you can sample a wide range of vegetarian dishes. Many of these groups also organize get-togethers for special events, such as Fourth of July picnics or Thanksgiving dinners.

These meetings are a good place to discuss such topics as where to find good vegetarian food in your neighborhood, how to handle sticky situations with nonvegetarian family members and friends, what to fix to eat for holiday meals and how to entertain guests, and to share other ideas about living a vegetarian lifestyle.

To find a vegetarian organization in your community, check your local phone book or inquire at your neighborhood natural foods store. You might also check with a national vegetarian organization to see if it knows of an active group near you. If you have no vegetarian groups in your area, you might consider starting one yourself. A national organization such as the Vegetarian Resource Group can assist you with materials and advice.

# Where to Go for More Information

There is an abundance of great resources for vegetarians, including books, cookbooks, periodicals, national organizations, and on-line contacts. Check out vegetarian books and cookbooks at your local library or bookstore.

## Periodicals

*Issues in Vegetarian Dietetics.* Quarterly newsletter of Vegetarian Nutrition, a dietetic practice group of The American Dietetic Association. Write to DPG #14, Division of Practice, The American Dietetic Association, 216 West Jackson Blvd., Chicago, IL 60606-6995, or call 1-312-899-0040 for information.

*Vegetarian Journal,* published bimonthly by the Vegetarian Resource Group, P.O. Box 1463, Baltimore, MD 21203, or call 1-410-366-VEGE.

*Veggie Life* magazine, EGW Publishing Company, 1041 Shary Circle, Concord, CA 94518, or call 1-510-671-9852 for more information.

*Vegetarian Times* magazine. P.O. Box 420235, Palm Coast, FL 32142-0235, or call 1-800-829-3340 for subscription orders and information.

## Organizations

### National Center for Nutrition and Dietetics

216 West Jackson Blvd.
Chicago, IL 60606-6995

The NCND is the public education center of The American Dietetic Association. To receive a free copy of the brochure, *Eating Well—The Vegetarian Way,* or a copy of *Fact Sheet: Vegetarian Diets,* send a self-addressed stamped envelope with your request to the address above. Callers can speak with registered dietitians regarding specific nutrition questions by calling the Center's consumer hot line at 1-900-225-5267. Referrals to registered dietitians nationwide are also available by calling 1-800-366-1655.

**Vegetarian Resource Group**
P.O. Box 1463
Baltimore, MD 21203
1-410-366-VEGE
   The VRG is a national, nonprofit vegetarian educational organization that publishes the bimonthly *Vegetarian Journal* as well as pamphlets, books, and other materials. Write or call for a catalog.

**North American Vegetarian Society**
P.O. Box 72
Dolgeville, NY 13329
1-518-568-7970
   The NAVS sponsors the annual Vegetarian Summerfest. Write or call for more details.

**Seventh Day Adventist Dietetic Association**
P.O. Box 75
Loma Linda, CA 92354

## Resources on the Internet

**Veggies Unite!** features vegetarian recipes and other information. The web address is: http://www.vegweb.com/

**Vegetarian Pages** is a worldwide Internet guide for vegetarian and vegan information. The web address is: http://www.veg.org/veg/

**The Vegetarian Resource Group** provides information on vegetarian diets as well as back issues of *Vegetarian Journal*. The web address is: http://www.vrg.org/

Also note that commercial on-line services such as America Online have user interest groups with vegetarian sections.

# Glossary

**Antioxidants** Substances in food that help fight infection and disease by protecting cells from the harmful effects of oxidation. Vitamins C, E, and beta carotene are antioxidants.

**Falafel** Small, deep-fried patties made from a mashed garbanzo bean mixture and often eaten in a pita pocket; Middle Eastern.

**Hummus** A Middle Eastern dip made from garbanzo beans.

**Lacto-ovo vegetarian** A person who avoids meat, fish, and poultry but may eat eggs and dairy products.

**Lacto-vegetarian** A person who avoids meat, fish, and poultry but may eat dairy products, such as milk, cheese, and yogurt. Lacto-vegetarians also avoid eggs and any foods that contain eggs or egg derivatives.

**Meat-restrictors** A person who avoids red meat but eats fish and poultry.

**Millet** A tiny, round yellow grain; a good source of zinc.

**Miso** A Japanese fermented soy paste often used to make soups; a good source of zinc.

**Phytochemicals** Non-nutrient compounds in food that help protect against infection and disease. Small amounts occur naturally in fruits, vegetables, herbs, and grains.

**Seitan** A wheat gluten product that can replace meat in recipes.

**Semi-vegetarian** A person who avoids red meat but eats fish and poultry.

**Spanakopita** A Greek spinach pie.

**Swiss chard** An iron-rich dark green leafy vegetable.

**Tempeh** A soybean cake held together by a mold culture.

**Textured vegetable protein (TVP)** A meat replacer made of soy protein. TVP granules absorb fluid and acquire the chewy consistency of meat.

**Tahini** Sesame butter; a good source of calcium.

**Tofu** Soybean curd; a good source of calcium.

**Vegan** A person who avoids all animal products.

**Vegetable paella** A traditional Spanish rice dish.

# Index